Beating Neuropathy

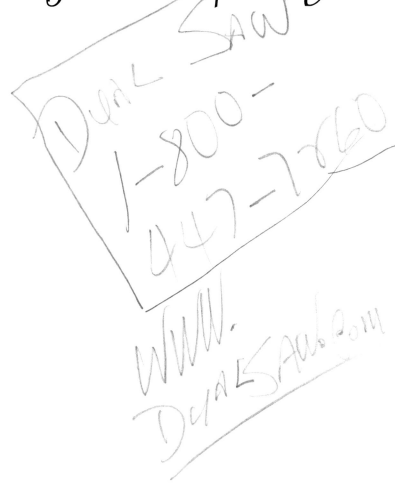

Dual Saw
1-800-
447-7760

WWW.
DualSaw.com

Beating Neuropathy

Taking Misery to Miracles in Just 5 Weeks

DR. JOHN HAYES JR.

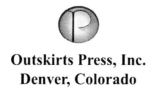

Outskirts Press, Inc.
Denver, Colorado

Beating Neuropathy
Taking Misery to Miracles in Just 5 Weeks
All Rights Reserved.
Copyright © 2010 Dr. John Hayes Jr.
V3.0

Outskirts Press, Inc.
http://www.outskirtspress.com

ISBN: 978-1-4327-4897-5

Outskirts Press and the "OP" logo are trademarks belonging to Outskirts Press, Inc.

Table of Contents

Dedication

This book is dedicated to the patients I have been fortunate enough to meet and work with throughout my career, who have been a continued source of inspiration. These are extraordinary people who have overcome extraordinary odds, yet still manage a smile and words of encouragement for myself and my team on a daily basis.

Now, I have the distinct pleasure and honor of bringing the successes in my practice to many more patients around the world. It is to you, my patients, that this book is dedicated.

About Dr. John Hayes, Jr.

Since 1981, in Private Practice specializing in successful multidisciplinary Healthcare with a focus on integrated case management, Dr. Hayes has an extensive clinically balanced background, and still works actively with many MDs, DMDs, DPMs PTs DCs PAs RNs, and others whose sole purpose is to deliver excellence in patient care. Dr. Hayes takes the time to really understand the problems and lifestyle of the patients we serve, and expects the same clinical excellence of his professional clients and students.

He is the founder of Health Solutions Group, treating patients using the staffing solutions and platforms we advocate in this book. Answers on personal patient care are found at www.neuropathydr. com

Our client doctors and students but especially our happiest patients know that Life Long health rests on a balance of regular professional care, proper nutrition, fitness programs, stress management, as well as mental health, with an emphasis on preventive healthcare.

As Practitioners, the challenge is to deliver this care in a manner that provides for our own wellbeing as well as the time and energy to enjoy our lives. Third party payers and regulatory bodies have made this evermore challenging.

Dr. Hayes' main purpose now is to provide fellow healthcare practitioners with the systems, platforms, tools and executive skills needed in today's very complex arena, without unneeded stress.

Information about this unique approach for patients, doctors, and other healthcare professionals may be found by registering at http://neuropathydr.com.

Preface

About Beating Peripheral Neuropathy

"I haven't slept well at all and the burning and tingling is just miserable. Nothing seems to help for long. It really hurts, plus I feel tired and groggy all the time from the medication…"

These are the some of the most common things patients say when afflicted with peripheral neuropathy. Neuropathy is really just your doctor's word for nerve "damage." It can be caused by many things, most commonly from unknown causes. Or it could be diabetes, chemotherapy, smoking, prescription medication and perhaps even over-the-counter self medication and dietary supplements. The more I work with neuropathy patients, the more the list really seems to go on and on.

Oftentimes, even brilliant physicians really can't find out exactly what causes some patients neuropathy.

But, the good news is that there is very significant progress being made in the treatment of peripheral neuropathy that now allows patients to not only get excellent in-office care, but to be discharged in a very reasonable period of time to a home treatment program with follow-up.

On the following pages, you will read more about my experiences using a combination of my many years of clinical practice since 1981 as well as the training, expertise and experience of a great man, Dr. David Phillips. David is the inventor of many medical devices (including the tympanic [ear] thermometer) and also the founder of ReBuilder Medical.

I was fortunate enough to find David when I was conducting research for my consulting clients on less cumbersome and more effective ways of treating the peripheral neuropathy patient in their offices. David has been an incredible wealth of knowledge and has assembled an incredible team of human beings, totally dedicated to *YOU*. You'll read much more about him as this story continues.

I also personally invite you to go to http://neuropathydr.com. We'll keep you up to date on our system advances, research and clinical studies as they expand.

Foreword for Your Doctor

Throughout my career and now with increasing frequency, I have had occasion to treat patients with peripheral neuropathy, with varying success. While consulting with other doctors, I discovered some were still very frustrated with their results treating peripheral neuropathy as well.

I began researching alternatives to current therapies, and was fortunate to find David Phillips, PhD. He is the inventor of many medical devices such as the tympanic thermometer and is the founder of ReBuilder Medical.

Upon my first conversation which ended up being about 2 hours, Dr. Phillips was kind enough to discuss with me at great length his use of his neuropathy treatment device, called the ReBuilder, which is a dual-frequency neuro-stimulator.

As our conversation continued, David and I discussed combining the ReBuilder neuro-stimulator with other therapies for neuropathy. Come to find out, David had already explored this aspect as well and had been employing some excellent biochemical methodologies in the treatment of peripheral neuropathy.

I was literally blown away by David's extensive knowledge of spinal mechanics and somatic dysfunction, as well as the neurology and pathophysiology that take place in peripheral neuropathy. He knows his neurophysiology and biochemistry better than many professors I have studied under.

I was fascinated that right before me was a device that had been the missing link to solving many months of misery and suffering that my patients had been reporting to me for over 20 years.

David and I continued our conversation and discussed a combined treatment protocol using not only his devices but chiropractic spinal manipulation, joint mobilization, and other mechanical therapies such as massage, stretching and exercise, as well as our combined years of experience with therapeutic nutrition.

A very short time later, I put together a treatment protocol using both of our inputs. Within the next six weeks I was absolutely astounded, not only with the results I had achieved in the office but also by how many people responded to our notices that we now had powerful and effective care for a condition that devastates the health and wellbeing of over 20 million Americans.

What I'd like to do next is give you just a brief synopsis of some case studies. To the best of my knowledge, this is the first time that a comprehensive outpatient drug-free treatment program has ever proven to be so effective, so quickly.

The first patient is an 80-year-old lady who presented in my office with a long history of diabetes. She had been diabetic for about 10 years and was suffering so badly from peripheral neuropathy that she had been unable to sleep for four years.

She was complaining primarily of burning, tingling, very significant sleep disturbance and a complete loss of sensation in her left great toe, which obviously was very annoying and interfering with her gait, thus aggravating her lower back.

When I performed her initial sensory examination, I found she had complete loss of sensation to light touch and vibration in her left great toe. She also had decreased sensation to touch and vibration along the lateral aspects and dorsum of both feet, but not the total loss that was shown on the left side.

Four sessions into her first 5-week trial using this new treatment protocol in the office, she started to experience sensation in her great toe. To make a long story very short, in five weeks this patient was discharged to a home-treatment program and continues to do very well.

It's very important to note that with this patient, my very first using this protocol, after her second week of treatment she was sleeping through the night every night except for one, and reported almost no peripheral neuropathy symptoms. She had had absolutely phenomenal results. Needless to say, I was blown away.

A short time later, there presented to my office one of the most challenging cases I have ever seen. This lady was a 53-year-old who presented with her husband, in a wheelchair.

At age 47 she was diagnosed with cervical cancer, which was cured. However, during her cancer care she was treated with cisplatin, which is as you know very potent neurotoxin.

When we did her examination, obviously she had a very difficult time ambulating because of the complete loss of sensation from her hips to her toes. When we did her sensory examination, she had no sensation to light touch from the hips down. Her feet were literally ice cold. Her legs were pale. She had no vibration sensation at all anywhere distal to the iliac crest (from her hips down to her toes).

Learning what I could from Dr. Phillips, I decided that this would be a very good test case to take in. I'm certainly glad I did because five weeks into treatment, I helped her walk down the hall without assistance. She did need a crutch, but this was the first time in many months that she had been able to ambulate without assistance. It was absolutely unbelievable. This woman had been in a wheelchair for four years.

The next patient was an amazing chemotherapy patient as well. This lady was a 54-year-old accountant. Unfortunately, she had colon cancer at a very young age and was treated with mixed chemotherapies. Her treatment included radiation, colostomy and, ultimately, surgical reversal of the colostomy.

She had a great outcome and her cancer was cured. Following the cancer treatment, however, she was left with peripheral neuropathy involving both hands and feet.

She presented to my office as a patient with a more classic type of stocking-and-glove neuropathy, complaining of tingling as well as sleep disturbance. At the time of her initial presentation, she was taking the prescription medication Lyrica, which did give her some softening of her symptoms, but no great alleviation.

After beginning our treatment protocol, she started to get the sensation back in her feet. At two weeks, not only had her peripheral neuropathy symptoms improved, her skin temperatures and textures had as well. In addition to having restoration of more normal sensation to her feet, she began to experience restoration of sensation to her hands.

Doctors and patients alike would have to agree that these cases are nothing short of miraculous. Previously, treating peripheral neuropathy patients hasn't been really successful. Often, it has been hit or miss. We've had some pretty good results in the past with nutrition therapy and I know other doctors are treating neuropathy patients with different combined modalities, but I've never seen resolutions like I've seen in these cases.

Furthermore, I have never seen another system that is so easy to use, easy to train the patient in and fosters patient independence from professional in-office care.

These cases obviously highlight the need for more research, which I'm happy to announce is ongoing and expanding interdisciplinary at an exponential rate.

Meanwhile, it's most important to me right now that more doctors learn how to help patients with peripheral neuropathy.

To that end, I have produced physicians education, training and support on this breakthrough treatment system. You can access the physicians support materials and learn more about this FDA and Medicare approved device at http://rebuildermedical.com, and connect with treating doctors and physical therapists at http://neuropathydr.com

1

What is Peripheral Neuropathy?

Peripheral neuropathy describes a condition that is characterized by some or all of the following: loss of sensation, tingling, numbness and burning, sleep disturbance and all the other unpleasant sensations that patients who have been diagnosed with peripheral neuropathy (PN) experience.

Peripheral neuropathy is very widespread. It has been estimated that somewhere between 15 million and 20 million patients suffer from it in the United States alone.

It has also been estimated that the annual costs of treating peripheral neuropathy in the United States alone are phenomenal. One study discovered that the complications from diabetic peripheral neuropathy alone approach $11 billion! The total cost of diabetic peripheral neuropathy and its complications is really extraordinary, approaching $14 billion annually. Up to 27% of the direct medical costs of diabetes may be attributed to diabetic peripheral neuropathy.

If you like, you can personally do up to the minute research on the treatment of virtually any health condition, including neuropathy on line.

You'll find the traditional, the fringe, the alternatives, and it really can be dizzying.

You like most patients have likely done so already.

You can also go to the National Library of Medicine on-line http://ncbi.nlm.nih.gov/**pubmed**/ or do a literature search on any search engine and find many references.

However, we have found our patients do best initially to connect with a licensed health care professional trained in the use of this system, and to sort through the clutter. And we help keep all of them up to date, so you don't have to.

2

What Can Cause
Peripheral Neuropathy?

The causes of peripheral neuropathy are in many cases unfortunately unknown. In fact, the most common cause of neuropathy in this day and age may actually be what's called idiopathic, meaning of unknown certainty. It's no longer diabetes.

In our modern world, we are subjected and exposed to many environmental toxins, including heavy metals. We also are seeing patients surviving cancer and living much longer. Unfortunately, one of the undesired complications of chemotherapy is the development of peripheral neuropathy. We are also seeing patients developing compression neuropathy, such as carpal tunnel, chronic sciatica and back pain and nerve damage associated with conditions like degenerative spinal disc disease and spinal stenosis. Part of this, of course, is because we are living longer and being more active than ever before.

Another common but often overlooked cause of peripheral neuropathy is the use of statin medication, which has expanded exponentially. It's not too long ago that the statins were heralded to be the cure-all for many of mankind's greatest diseases and illnesses. This is not the forum to debate the appropriate use of statins but if you or family members are taking them, you do need to be aware that peripheral neuropathy is a potential complication.

There are other causes of peripheral neuropathy, like kidney disease and hormonal diseases that occur in patients with hyperthyroidism, as well as Cushing's disease, which affects the adrenal glands and the output of cortisol.

Alcoholism can cause peripheral neuropathy, as can vitamin deficiencies, especially deficiencies of thiamin, or vitamin B1. There are still more causes: chronic hypertension, cigarette-smoking, immune-complex diseases, generalized degenerative lifestyles that include obesity, poor diet combined with cigarette smoking, abuse of over-the-counter medications, etc.

Whatever your condition, it is important to work with your entire healthcare team, preferably with just one professional in charge. This may very well be your MD, DC or PT in charge. Avoid unnecessary duplication of tests. Make sure everybody knows about medication usage, supplement usage, and any personal changes in your health history.

Until our healthcare system finally has centralized records, help your doctor by keeping copies of all your records and test results in one location, providing them to your doctors when you present for your initial evaluation.

3

How Do I Know If I Have Peripheral Neuropathy?

Knowing if you have peripheral neuropathy should be very straightforward.

Unfortunately, patients with peripheral neuropathy suffer greatly. In my experience and the experience of many physicians, patients have symptoms for years, which gradually build to a crescendo before they present to our offices.

These symptoms initially may include such things as mild loss of sensation of the hands and the feet, progressive worsening of tingling and numbness that will oftentimes wake the patient at night, or completely disturbed sleep.

We also find that many patients with peripheral neuropathy have a combination of these most annoying symptoms. This could include not only the presence of tingling and numbness but shooting pains. I have had many patients tell me that one of the most annoying symptoms, especially in colder climates, is the coolness of the feet as well as the (trophic) changes that occur in the skin. Sometimes, that is extreme dryness, cracking, fragility etc.

The diagnosis of peripheral neuropathy really is a diagnosis of exclusion. I tell my doctors this all the time. It is very important to have a doctor working with you, who is able to perform the most thorough physical evaluation possible, evaluate all of your medical records to make sure that all correctible causes of peripheral neuropathy have been addressed. If a root cause can be identified it should be addressed as completely as is medically and humanly possible.

A diagnosis of peripheral neuropathy is more about making sure of everything it's not. Therefore, our client doctors who take care of peripheral neuropathy patients commonly work with many physicians of other disciplines. The reasons for this should be quite obvious. It is very important that all the things we spoke about earlier, such as family history, genetics, medication usage, etc are all accounted for.

We also have to be on the lookout for iatrogenically caused neuropathy from medical care such as chemotherapy for cancer or other illnesses.

Another area which concerns me greatly is when patients self-medicate with over-the-counter medications or maybe even herbal preparations that possibly could be contaminated with heavy metals or plant toxins.

I strongly advise you to seek professional counseling before creating irreversible damage to your liver or kidneys.

4

Are All the Peripheral Neuropathies the Same?

No. All the peripheral neuropathies are not the same. We find, though, that the patients who present with peripheral neuropathy, regardless of the cause, do have remarkably similar symptoms.

The good news with our treatment program has been that even in the presence of similar symptoms from different etiologies (causes), the corrective care for is often remarkably effective regardless of the primary cause. That is the beauty of the treatment system that we have been able to employ.

In order to find out what components of peripheral neuropathy you have, your doctor will conduct a very thorough evaluation. This will include things such as your vital signs, body mass index, the mobility and range of motion of your lower back and hips, and the overall health of your feet, skin, nails and hair, blood vessels and circulation. This might include doppler ultrasound, a simple painless test to check for blood flow or blockages.

As the doctor performs her clinical examination, she'll also perform a very thorough neurological examination including reflexes, muscle-testing, and sensation to touch using a device as simple as a pin, a brush or perhaps even a pinwheel. Doctors commonly will also check your vibration sensation, which very often is disturbed in peripheral neuropathy. This is done painlessly and very easily through the use of simple tuning forks. Your balance will be assessed.

Laboratory tests may very well be performed. These would include things such as a chemistry panel, kidney and liver function. Your doctor will also want to double check your blood sugar levels and more than likely perform a hemoglobin A1c.

This particular test is very good at identifying patients who may be borderline diabetic. I have found many patients who present with neuropathy symptoms have not yet been diagnosed with diabetes but may very well suffer from what's called metabolic syndrome.

There is some very understandable patient information on this here: http://en.wikipedia.org/wiki/Metabolic_syndrome and your bodies abnormal handling of blood sugar, which may unfortunately lead to the development of neuropathy and other diabetic complications **well before** the formal diagnosis is made. You and Your healthcare professionals need to be aware of this research as well, two of the best synopses from the National Library of Medicine which are on-line at Pub Med http://pubmed.gov and are reprinted here:

1: J Neurol Sci. 2006 Mar 15;242(1-2):9-14. Epub 2006 Jan 30.

Idiopathic neuropathy, prediabetes and the metabolic syndrome.

Gordon Smith A, Robinson Singleton J.

Neurology and Pathology, University of Utah School of Medicine, 30 North 1900 East, SOM 3R152, Salt Lake City, UT 84132, USA. Gordon.smith@hsc.utah.edu

Peripheral neuropathy is a common problem encountered by neurologists and primary care physicians. While there are many causes for peripheral neuropathy, none can be identified in a large percentage of patients ("idiopathic neuropathy"). Despite its high prevalence, idiopathic neuropathy is poorly studied and understood. There is evolving evidence that impaired glucose tolerance (prediabetes) is associated with idiopathic neuropathy. Preliminary data from a multicenter study of diet and exercise in prediabetes (the Impaired Glucose Tolerance Neuropathy Study) suggests a diet and exercise counseling regimen based on the Diabetes Prevention Program results in improved metabolic measures and small fiber function. Prediabetes is part of the Metabolic Syndrome, which also includes hypertension, hyperlipidemia and obesity. Individual aspects of the Metabolic Syndrome influence risk and progression of diabetic neuropathy and may play a causative role in neuropathy both for those with prediabetes, and those with otherwise idiopathic neuropathy. Thus, a multifactorial treatment approach to individual components of Metabolic Syndrome may slow prediabetic neuropathy progression or result in improvement.

PMID: 16448668 [PubMed - indexed for MEDLINE

1: Am J Manag Care. 2008 Dec;14(12):791-8.

Complications of dysglycemia and medical costs associated with nondiabetic hyperglycemia.

Nichols GA, Arondekar B, Herman WH.

Center for Health Research, Kaiser Permanente, Portland, OR 97227-1098, USA. greg.nichols@kpchr.org

OBJECTIVE: To estimate the prevalence of complications associated with diabetes in patients with hyperglycemia below the threshold for diabetes, and to evaluate the associated medical costs. STUDY DESIGN: Retrospective observational cohort study. METHODS: We used fasting and random glucose test results, and a previously validated predictive equation to assign 26,111 nondiabetic patients to the following categories: normoglycemia, isolated impaired fasting glucose (I-IFG), isolated impaired glucose tolerance (I-IGT), or IFG with IGT (IFG/IGT). We identified microvascular complications (retinopathy, neuropathy, nephropathy) and macrovascular complications (cardiovascular disease, stroke, peripheral vascular disease, heart failure) commonly associated with diabetes from electronic medical records. We then calculated and compared the impacts of hyperglycemia and its complications in terms of age/sex-adjusted mean annual medical care costs. RESULTS: Complications were most prevalent among the I-IGT and IFG/IGT patients -- more than half (51.1% in each group) had at least 1 complication compared with 33.9% of normoglycemic patients (P <.001 for both comparisons). Macrovascular complications added $3,863 (P <.0001) to annual age/sex-adjusted per-person medical costs; microvascular complications added $1,874 (P <.0001). I-IGT ($716; P <.0001) and IFG/IGT ($438; P = .009) independently added to costs after controlling for presence of any complication. CONCLUSIONS: For many patients, complications associated with hyperglycemia appear to develop before diabetes diagnosis. Complications add significantly to the cost of medical care at hyperglycemic levels below the threshold for diabetes. However, the increased prevalence of complications did not completely explain the observed differences in age/sex-adjusted medical care costs.

PMID: 19067496 [PubMed - indexed for MEDLINE]

You can help your doctor along by bringing copies of laboratory tests that may have been performed within the couple of years prior to your office visit. In this day and age especially, it's very important that diagnostic tests that have already been performed are not duplicated unnecessarily.

Additional considerations in diagnosing peripheral neuropathy include the application of things like NCV, or nerve conduction velocities. These are oftentimes performed in the offices of neurologists and other healthcare providers who are trained and certified in their application.

The good news is that there are also other items on the horizon that will make the measurements of nerve conduction velocity much easier and more straightforward, and these will be applied to the studies that are ongoing in our patients that suffer from peripheral neuropathy.

Something else that really affects all peripheral neuropathy patients is that drug only treatment to date has been of very limited effectiveness.

Patients oftentimes try many drugs, costing many hundreds of dollars out of their own pockets that prove to ultimately be ineffective.

Nutrition therapy may be part of the answer, but is not the entire answer.

I say this not only from my own personal experience, but also from the experience of other doctors I've consulted with and from speaking with my patients over the years.

In fact, as I stated earlier, one of the worst things that can happen is when a patient attempts to treat his or her own peripheral neuropathy **without** the guidance of a trained and licensed healthcare professional.

Here are just a few more synopses direct from Pub Med to help educate you and your doctor on the role of nutrients in managing peripheral neuropathy:

1: Exp Clin Endocrinol Diabetes. 1999;107(7):421-30.Links

Alpha-lipoic acid in the treatment of diabetic polyneuropathy in Germany: current evidence from clinical trials.

Ziegler D, Reljanovic M, Mehnert H, Gries FA.

Diabetes-Forschungsinstitut an der Heinrich-Heine-Universität, Düsseldorf, Germany. dan.ziegler@dfi.uni-duesseldorf.de

Diabetic neuropathy represents a major health problem, as it is responsible for substantial morbidity, increased mortality, and impaired quality of life. Near-normoglycaemia is now generally accepted as the primary approach to prevention of diabetic neuropathy, but is not achievable in a considerable number of patients. In the past two decades several medical treatments that exert their effects despite hyperglycaemia have been derived from the experimental pathogenetic concepts of diabetic neuropathy. Such compounds have been designed to improve or slow the progression of the neuropathic process and are being evaluated in clinical trials, but with the exception of alpha-lipoic acid (thioctic acid) which is available in Germany, none of these drugs is currently available in clinical practice. Here we review the current evidence from the clinical trials that assessed the therapeutic efficacy and safety of thioctic acid in diabetic polyneuropathy. Thus far, 15 clinical trials have been completed using different study designs, durations of treatment, doses, sample sizes, and patient populations. Within this variety of clinical trials, those with beneficial effects of thioctic acid on either neuropathic symptoms and deficits due to polyneuropathy or reduced heart rate variability resulting from cardiac autonomic neuropathy used doses of at least 600 mg per day. The following conclusions can be drawn from the recent controlled clinical trials. 1.) Short-term treatment for 3 weeks using 600 mg of thioctic acid i.v. per day appears to reduce the chief symptoms of diabetic polyneuropathy. A 3-week pilot study of 1800 mg per day given orally indicates that the therapeutic effect may be independent of the route of administration, but this needs to be confirmed in a larger sample size. 2.) The effect on symptoms is accompanied by an improvement of neuropathic deficits. 3.) Oral treatment for 4-7 months tends to reduce neuropathic deficits and improves cardiac autonomic neuropathy. 4.) Preliminary data over 2 years indicate possible long-term improvement in motor and sensory nerve conduction in the lower limbs. 5.) Clinical and postmarketing surveillance studies have revealed a highly favourable safety profile of the drug. Based on these findings, a pivotal long-term multicenter trial of oral treatment with thioctic acid (NATHAN I Study) is being conducted in North America and Europe aimed at slowing the progression of diabetic polyneuropathy using a clinically meaningful and reliable primary outcome measure that combines clinical and neurophysiological assessment.

PMID: 10595592 [PubMed - indexed for MEDLINE]

1: Exp Clin Endocrinol Diabetes. 2008 Nov;116(10):600-5. Epub 2008 May 13.

Benfotiamine in diabetic polyneuropathy (BENDIP): results of a randomised, double blind, placebo-controlled clinical study.

Stracke H, Gaus W, Achenbach U, Federlin K, Bretzel RG.

Medical Clinic und Policlinic III, University Hospital Giessen and Marburg, Location Giessen, Germany. Hilmar.Stracke@innere.med. uni-giessen.de

AIM: Efficacy and safety of benfotiamine in treatment of diabetic polyneuropathy. METHODS: Double blind, placebo-controlled, phase-III-study. 181 patients were screened. 165 patients with symmetrical, distal diabetic polyneuropathy were randomised to one of three treatment groups entering the wash-out phase and 133/124 patients were analysed in the ITT/PP analysis: Benfotiamine 600 mg per day (n=47/43), benfotiamine 300 mg per day (n=45/42) or placebo (n=41/39). RESULTS: After 6 weeks of treatment, the primary outcome parameter NSS (Neuropathy Symptom Score) differed significantly between the treatment groups (p=0.033) in the PP (per protocol) population. In the ITT (intention to treat) population, the improvement of NSS was slightly above significance (p=0.055). The TSS (Total Symptom Score) showed no significant differences after 6 weeks of treatment. The improvement was more pronounced at the higher benfotiamine dose and increased with treatment duration. In the TSS, best results were obtained for the symptom "pain". Treatment was well tolerated in all groups. CONCLUSION: Benfotiamine may extend the treatment option for patients with diabetic polyneuropathy based on causal influence on impaired glucose metabolism. Further studies should confirm the positive experiences.

PMID: 18473286 [PubMed - indexed for MEDLINE]

Related articles

Benfotiamine in the treatment of diabetic polyneuropathy--a three-week randomized, controlled pilot study (BEDIP study).

Int J Clin Pharmacol Ther. 2005 Feb; 43(2):71-7.

[Int J Clin Pharmacol Ther. 2005]

Treatment of symptomatic diabetic polyneuropathy with the antioxidant alpha-lipoic acid: a 7-month multicenter randomized controlled trial (ALADIN III Study). ALADIN III Study Group. Alpha-Lipoic Acid in Diabetic Neuropathy.

Diabetes Care. 1999 Aug; 22(8):1296-301.

[Diabetes Care. 1999]

Treatment of symptomatic diabetic polyneuropathy with the antioxidant alpha-lipoic acid: a meta-analysis.

Diabet Med. 2004 Feb; 21(2):114-21.

[Diabet Med. 2004]

Treatment of diabetic polyneuropathy with the antioxidant thioctic acid (alpha-lipoic acid): a two year multicenter randomized double-blind placebo-controlled trial (ALADIN II). Alpha Lipoic Acid in Diabetic Neuropathy.

Free Radic Res. 1999 Sep; 31(3):171-9.

[Free Radic Res. 1999]

Review

Repaglinide : a pharmacoeconomic review of its use in type 2 diabetes mellitus.

Pharmacoeconomics. 2004; 22(6):389-411.

[Pharmacoeconomics. 2004]

Patient Drug Information

Thiamine is a vitamin used by the body to break down sugars in the diet. The medication helps correct nerve and heart problems that occur when a person's diet does not contain enough thiamine.

: <u>Ann Pharmacother.</u> 2008 Nov;42(11):1686-91. Epub 2008 Oct 21.

Role of acetyl-L-carnitine in the treatment of diabetic peripheral neuropathy.

Evans JD, **Jacobs TF**, **Evans EW**.

Department of Clinical and Administrative Sciences, College of Pharmacy, University of Louisiana at Monroe, Monroe, LA, USA. jevans@ulm.edu

OBJECTIVE: To examine the role of acetyl-L-carnitine (ALC) in the treatment of diabetic peripheral neuropathy (DPN). DATA SOURCES: A MEDLINE search (1966-April 2008) of the English-language literature was performed using the search terms carnitine, diabetes, nerve, and neuropathy. Studies identified were then cross-referenced for their citations. STUDY SELECTION AND DATA EXTRACTION: The search was limited to clinical trials, meta-analyses, and reviews addressing the use of ALC for the treatment of DPN. Studies that included other disease states that could cause peripheral neuropathy were excluded. Two large clinical studies that used ALC for the treatment of DPN were identified. No case studies were identified. DATA SYNTHESIS: The results from 2 published clinical trials involving 1679 subjects were included. Subjects who received at least 2 g daily of ALC showed decreases in pain scores. One study showed improvements in electrophysiologic factors such as nerve conduction velocities, while the other did not. Patients who had neuropathic pain reported reductions in pain using a visual analog scale. Nerve regeneration was documented in one trial. The supplement was well tolerated. A proprietary form of ALC was used in both studies. CONCLUSIONS: Data on treatment of DPN with ALC support its use. It should be recommended to patients early in the disease process to provide maximal benefit. Further studies should be conducted to determine the effectiveness of ALC in the treatment and prevention of the worsening symptoms of DPN.

PMID: 18940920 [PubMed - indexed for MEDLINE]

1: Turk Neurosurg. 2007 Apr;17(2):67-77.

Neuroprotective effects of acetyl-L-carnithine in experimental chronic compression neuropathy. A prospective, randomized and placebo-control trials.

Kotil K, Kirali M, Eras M, Bilge T, Uzun H.

Haseki Educational and Research Hospital, Neurosurgery Clinic, Istanbul, Turkey. kadirkotil@superonline.com

OBJECTIVE: We designed this experimental study to examine the potential positive influences of the acetylated derivative of acetyl-L-carnithine, an endogenous substance present in the nervous system, on chronic compression neuropathy. This is the first study ever published on the medical treatment of experimental chronic compression neuropathy. MATERIALS AND METHODS: Five groups composed of 5 rats each were used in the study. Group 1: The control group, in which a 1 cm-long segment proximally from the bifurcation point of the right sciatic nerve of each rat was excised, accompanied by removal of the right soleus muscle. Group 2: The compression neuropathy model group, in which the right sciatic nerve of each rat was compressed for 30 days. Group 3: The right sciatic nerves were compressed for 30 days, followed by decompression and assessment on the 60th day. Group 4: The right sciatic nerves were compressed for 30 days, followed by decompression and acetyl-Lcarnithine administration between days 30 and 60. Group 5: The right sciatic nerves were compressed for 30 days, followed by acetyl-L-carnithine administration from day 30 to 60 without decompression. The study continued with the rats in the other 3 groups. Rats in the 3rd group were treated with decompression only and kept for another 1 month. Rats in the 4th group received acetyl-L-carnithine at a dose of 20 mg/kg/day intraperitoneally for 1 month after decompression, whereas rats in the 5th group received only intraperitoneal acetyl-L-carnithine at a dose of 20 mg/kg/day without decompression. Like the rats in groups 1 and 2, these rats were also sacrificed with ether overdose, with their right sciatic nerves and soleus muscles being excised for histopathological examination and weighing, respectively. CONCLUSION: In our study, it was found that decompression significantly improves the recovery rate of peripheral nerve as compared with that without decompression, and that acetyl-L-carnithine coadministered with decompression enhances clinical and histopathological recovery. In addition, the use of silicon tubes in such experiments was found to be likely to have prominent advantages.

PMID: 17935020 [PubMed - indexed for MEDLINE]

5

What's the Common Link in the Neuropathies?

This is the most amazing part that I have discovered in my work with Dr. David Phillips. The common link in all of these peripheral neuropathies, regardless of the cause, appears to be hypoxia.

Hypoxia is simply a word that describes loss of oxygen. This occurs at what are called the neuronal junctions. That is, the areas in the human body where one nerve cell communicates to another.

At a simplistic level, nerve cells communicate electrochemically across a gap. In neuropathy caused by hypoxia, this neuronal gap widens, which is theorized to be responsible for the symptoms that include not only the burning and the tingling but the shooting pains as well.

I have with permission, reprinted some of Dr. Phillips work below:

Neuropathy and chronic pain: The Condition

By David Phillps, PhD

Neuropathy and chronic pain is characterized by pain, numbness, loss of tactile feedback, and poor tissue perfusion. These symptoms may indicate that oxygen is not getting to all the cells causing dysfunction.

Because the patient's quality of life is decreased, these results are often devastating. Pain medications do not cure the condition; it only helps mask it and, eventually, leads to complications with adverse side effects such as mental confusion and intestinal problems. As a result of conducting our own research and reviewing published studies from around the world, we have been led to new models concerning the causes of neuropathy and chronic pain. We have concluded that it is not reasonable to merely label neuropathy and chronic pain symptoms as diabetic, peripheral, vascular, or "idiopathic". What is needed is a more full understanding of the etiology of the condition so new technology can be brought to bear with both ameliorative and therapeutic benefits.

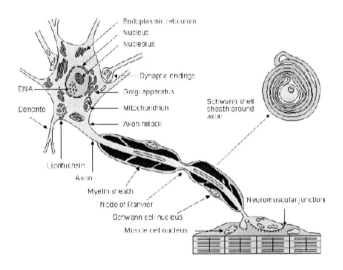

Figure 1: Anatomy of a nerve cell

Neuropathy and chronic pain results when nerve signal propagation is reduced between adjacent nerve cells due to insufficient oxygen being available to support nerve cell metabolism. This is responsible for 90% of all neuropathy and chronic pain cases. The remaining 10% is caused by physical trauma. Thus it appears that the main precipitating factor for neuropathy and chronic pain is hypoxia and demineralization of the synaptic fluid which creates shrinkage of the nerve cells which widens the gap between these cells making it more difficult for normal sensations to propagate, and loss of electrical conductivity in the synaptic fluid itself.

A temporary hypoxia of nerve tissue can be traced to most causes of neuropathy and chronic pain. The primary negative effects of this hypoxia are as follows:

- A defensive contraction of the nerve cell resulting in oversize synaptic junctions

- A loss of electrical conductivity of the synaptic fluid between nerve cells

- A defensive change in the electrical potentials of the cell membrane resulting in a higher resting state of the trigger level which effectively limits the sensitivity to incoming signals

For example, when the lumbar area experiences a muscle spasm, blood flow is restricted through that muscle resulting in reduced oxygen availability to the surrounding tissue, including nerve cells. Because muscles can use either oxygen or glucose metabolic pathways, they can recover quickly from a temporary reduction in the level of available oxygen. Nerve cells, on the other hand, are limited to the Krebs oxidative reductive metabolic system and must take immediate defensive steps to assure survival during this hypo oxygen state. One of the ways they accomplish this is to contract along their longitudinal axis like a rubber band, reducing their surface area and thus lowering their need for oxygen. (This also occurs when these cells are attacked by a harsh agent in the blood such as chemotherapeutic drugs, Agent Orange, environmental toxins, insecticides, etc.) The synaptic junctions between the axons of one nerve cell and the dendrites of the next nerve cell widen. Normal nerve transmission is now compromised because a nerve signal of normal intensity cannot jump this newly widened gap. The synaptic fluid between the nerve cells must be electrically conductive. Pure water does not conduct electricity, so this conductivity relies on minerals and specific neurotransmitters such as serotonin in the synaptic fluid to enable the propagation of the nerve signal. These minerals are delivered via the perfusion of adjacent tissues with fresh blood and kept in suspension by the periodic ionization of successfully transmitted nerve signals across the junction. When nerve signals are reduced because of these larger dimensions of the synaptic junction, necessary minerals are no longer held in place by electrical tension and are slowly leeched out.

(See Figure 2) This adds to the impairment of effective nerve transmission.

Common short term remedies with prescription drugs only ameliorate the pain temporarily and do little or nothing to mitigate or cure the underlying condition. They may provide some level of temporary relief, but as the disease progresses, the effective dosage of the drug needed to continue suppressing the pain

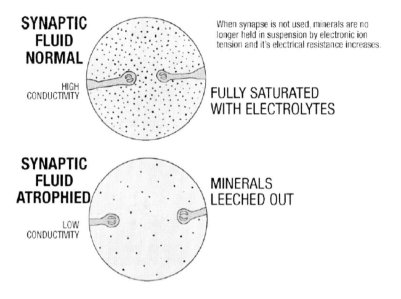

Figure 2: Minerals necessary for proper conduction across the synaptic junction can leech out when not actively used.

increases concurrently. The side effects of these types of drugs are difficult to deal with and add to the patient's discomfort. When the increased drug dosage reaches a threshold level, the patient can become confused, ataxic, constipated, confined to a wheelchair or may become bedridden. Symptoms similar to Alzheimer's may soon follow. When nerve signals can no longer jump the enlarged synaptic gap, the electrical tension that normally holds these minerals in place is absent, causing the synaptic fluid to leach out its mineral content. Electrical conductivity is reduced, thereby inhibiting the transmission of the normal nerves' electrical signals across this gap.

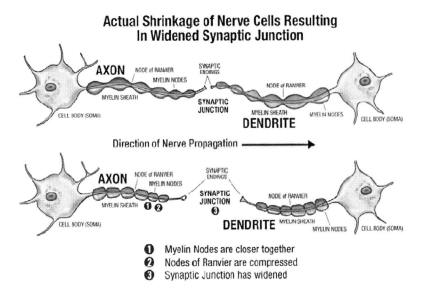

Figure 3: How a nerve cell shrinks resulting in a widened synaptic junction.

Neuropathy and chronic pain: the Causes

Trauma: Actual trauma is one of the major causes of neuropathy and chronic pain, and results when the myelin sheath is cut or etched away by chemotherapeutic agents, environmental toxins, poorly performed injections, or from amputations and accidents.

Traumatic causes must obviously be mitigated by removing the cause as in drug therapy, chemotherapy, physical entrapment, and environmental poisons. Permanent tissue damage may be beyond the scope of any therapy. When these conditions are removed, the ReBuilder® may be a helpful adjunctive therapy in the healing process.

Diabetes: Diabetes can also trigger neuropathy and chronic pain by affecting the levels of glucose and/or insulin in the blood stream. When this occurs, minerals are driven out of the fluid in the synaptic junction thereby reducing conductivity and impairing nerve impulse transmission. Nerve signals propagates from the cell body unidirectionally over the synapse, first along the axon and then across the synapse to the next nerve or muscle cell. The synaptic cleft, the gap between presynaptic terminal and postsynaptic terminal, has a thickness of 10 - 50 nm. The fact that the impulse transfers across the synapse only in one direction, from the presynaptic terminal to the postsynaptic terminal, is due to the difference in electrical polarity between the sending axon and the receiving dendrite. This is one of the reasons that the ReBuilder® sends its signal from one foot to the other – it sets the relative potential in each gap properly so that it forces the signal to jump properly, always toward the central nervous system and not miss-fire and jump the wrong way, perhaps to a sending axon that can lead to the periphery.

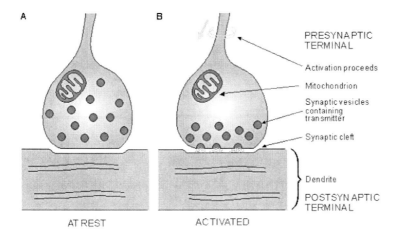

Figure 4 (A) At rest synaptic vesicles. (B) Activated synaptic vesicles (when activation reaches the presynaptic terminal, electrical signals jump across the synaptic cleft to activate the postsynaptic terminal).

As a result of hypoxic cellular atrophy, nerve signals must now try to jump a larger gap through a less conductive medium. This loss of nerve transmission is first perceived as tingling, then burning, and finally as pain when the demineralization and gap widening process progresses. The initial perception associated with atrophied nerves and enlarged synaptic gaps are tingling as some of the normal signals are misdirected to nearby nerves. As the condition progresses, it happens more and more until more signals are misdirected than properly happens propagated, and the resulting sensation is one of pain. Finally, after the nerve signals can no longer be transmitted at all, numbness is the primary complaint. This secondary effect of neuropathy and chronic pain reduces the strength of the calf muscles, which, in turn, reduces the blood flow to the lower extremities. This condition often results in poor tissue perfusion, insecure gait, balance problems, and other mobility issues.

Chemotherapeutic Agents: Prescribed for cancer precisely because they inhibit fast growing or fast acting cells, chemotherapeutic agents cause neuropathy and chronic pain in approximately one third of the patients to whom they are administered. Though nerve cells do not reproduce themselves like cancer cells do, they do change electrical states quickly and are thus particularly susceptible to the effects of chemotherapeutic drugs. The fast acting nerves are mistaken for fast growing neo-plasms. Chemotherapy has the effect of de-mineralizing the synaptic fluid, damaging the integrity of the nerve cells, and making it difficult for the ionization of the cell membranes to propagate the signal along the surface of the nerve. When ionization takes place, the outer membrane of the nerve cells change from positive to negative in a wave like motion taking a positive charge from one end of the nerve all the way to the other end. Chemotherapy is designed to interrupt the ability of the cell to control the permeability of the outer membrane and this process is electrically modulated. This electrical interruption is misapplied when the agent is in contact with the myelin sheath of a health, active nerve cell and causes the nerve cell to "short out" and inhibit the necessary different potentials in the nodes of the myelin sheath.

Cardiovascular Disease: By reducing the amount of blood that can perfuse the tissue of the lower legs and feet, cardiovascular disease can also cause neuropathy and chronic pain. When the arteries and veins become blocked, blood flow is reduced. One of the first symptoms is intermittent claudication which results in a reduction in the distance a patient can walk before the onset of localized leg pain due to reduced oxygen availability. Therefore, the muscle cells switch from aerobic metabolism to using anaerobic metabolism thereby creating greater than normal amounts of lactic acid, the by-product of muscle metabolism. The increased lactic acid collects in the cells causing inflammation and pain.

Lumbar Trauma: Trauma to the lumbar area of the back can be another cause of neuropathy and chronic pain. This trauma can be as slight as lifting a bag of groceries out of the trunk, picking up a grandchild, or bending down to tie a shoe. **Our studies show a 60% correlation between repeated injuries to the lower back and subsequent development of neuropathy and chronic pain symptoms.** (Emphasis added).

During the acute phase of localized trauma, inflammation develops reducing arterial and venous blood to the lumbar synaptic junctions. Nerves in the region temporarily shrink due to the reduction in activity. Since the body tends to conserve resources, the affected nerves begin to atrophy, the synaptic junction gap begins to widen, and synaptic minerals leech away making signal transmission more difficult.

Signals of normal strength can no longer cross synapses that are damaged by the reduction in blood flow. The loss of signals across the synapses compounds the process of deterioration.

Muscle atrophy and a host of other problems follow. We have found that a signal delivered at 7.83 cycles per second (the body's natural electromagnetic resonant frequency) and at an amplitude approximately 10 times that originally required will cross these enlarged synapses, repolarize them.

High Blood Pressure Medication: High blood pressure medication not only lowers blood pressure, it also reduces the ability of the arterial blood to refill the veins. This vacancy results as the venous muscle pumps the blood back to the heart. When this occurs the blood has a tendency to pool in the lower extremities; the nerves and synaptic junctions do not have enough necessary nutrition and oxygen to maintain their health resulting in nerve cell atrophy, loss of mineralization, and conductivity of the synaptic junctions as explained above.

Psychoactive Drug Therapy: These drugs, used to reduce anxiety or seizures, have the effect of reducing the intensity/frequency of all nerve signals. This, too, can result in loss of motor and sensory nerve function. These conditions can result in impaired mobility and balance issues due to the loss of muscle strength. Whenever overactive nerves that might be causing psychological problems are depressed, they depress borderline poorly functioning nerves as well.

Dr. Phillips brilliantly designed the device called the ReBuilder that seems clinically able to stimulate the nerves in such a way as to literally effect better "performance" at the neuronal junctions. By that I mean it actually appears that the neuronal gaps and junctions may be "closing".

It is quite likely that further research will enlighten us on exactly how this occurs but I believe that Dr. Phillips' device is very effective because it provides neuro-stimulation that literally "wakes up" and invokes repair to some extent of the nerve-"endings".

As you read from Dr. Phillips, Hypoxia can be caused by many situations that we experience throughout our lives. This loss of tissue oxygen could be due to trauma, or compression on a peripheral nerve such as can occur in the sciatic nerve at the hip and the lower back as well as the median nerve at the wrist and the ulnar nerve at the elbow. These last two conditions are called carpal tunnel syndrome and cubital tunnel syndrome respectively.

Unfortunately, patients with any of these conditions suffer greatly. The good news is that the combined methods of treatment that we'll be discussing may also be effective for these patients.

6

A 3-Part Solution for Rapid Change

We have discussed the causes of peripheral neuropathy and have in a very simplistic way addressed what might be actually occurring to cause nerve damage at the cellular level.

The good news is that we have been able to produce very effective treatments for peripheral neuropathies by combining three specific modalities.

The first is the application of manual therapy. Manual therapies, including massage, mobilization, stretching and spinal manipulation especially have been employed for centuries. The research literature abounds with the effectiveness of manual therapies for many conditions.

Despite abundant research, controversy of course still exists. However, I will tell you, as will any good doctor, that any treatment that proves to be cost-effective and is not harmful should be employed prior to the administration of more expensive and potentially harmful techniques such as powerful medications with unfortunate side effects.

The next part of the treatment protocol is nutrition therapy. This is something that really needs to be tailor-made. However, there are some nutrients that we should address in the context of discussing our treatment program for peripheral neuropathy.

The supplements that are used most commonly are prescribed by healthcare professionals only after the extensive evaluation is performed in the office. This would have to include, of course, all of your previous medical background, recent laboratory tests, as well as other tests that the doctor may determine warranted for your particular condition.

This is not a blanket recommendation for supplements, but I will address some of the more commonly prescribed supplements and the rationale for them.

Let's first of all talk about benfotiamine, which is actually synthetic vitamin B1. It turns out that benfotiamine has been used since the 1950s to treat alcoholic neuropathy, sciatica and other painful conditions in other countries around the world. Interestingly, benfotiamine is less toxic than a more commonly prescribed form of vitamin B1 called thiamine hydrochloride.

As far as I can determine from researching the literature, there have been no significant reports of adverse effects due to the use of vitamin B1 in the benfotiamine complex. The evidence certainly seems to suggest that there is a minimal downside to trying benfotiamine as part of a comprehensive treatment protocol.

Come to find out, one of the most brilliant things that Dr. Phillips did is incorporate the benfotiamine form in his dietary supplement called ReStore, one of the cornerstones of our 5-week treatment protocol.

There are a couple of other issues. One of the more common is managing the patient with diabetes. There are many dietary supplements that help patients with diabetes function better, feel better, have better exercise tolerance and ultimately manage their blood sugar better.

These particular supplements do need to be monitored by a licensed healthcare professional. This monitoring should include the patient's regular measurements of their fasting blood sugar levels, as well as periodic assessments of their hemoglobin A1c.

We commonly prescribe vitamin C, additional B vitamin complexes and chromium in the GTF form. The glucose tolerance factor form of chromium may help patients more easily regulate their blood sugar levels. This, combined with good advice from the doctor regarding exercise, weight-management, carbohydrate control etc, goes a long way to helping the diabetic patient with peripheral neuropathy.

There are also some other interesting dietary supplements that have been proven to help patients with peripheral neuropathy.

One of the most amazing substances is an amino acid called acetyl l-carnitine. In studies, Acetyl l-carnitine has proven not only to help neuropathic pain but also to assist in regeneration and vibratory perception. One of the most amazing things about it is that it helps to carry energy-producing molecules into cellular mitochondria.

The mitochondria are those portions of living nerve cells that are responsible for energy uptake. That may be one of the reasons that when these particular dietary supplements are combined with the other components of our program, patients experience such phenomenal results.

Other dietary supplements that may be used include antioxidants.

Antioxidants are molecules or compounds that are capable of slowing the oxidation of other molecules.

Oxidation is a chemical reaction that can produce damage through the formation of free radicals at the cellular level. Free-radical damage is responsible for damage to DNA, which can result in a wide variety of diseases, premature aging and so on.

It is impossible to stop oxidation in its entirety. However, it is very likely that better nutritional support can slow the oxidative processes that lead to premature aging, degeneration and unfortunately, the progression of peripheral neuropathy as well.

Here is more about our 3-part solution for managing peripheral neuropathies.

My early conversations with Dr. Phillips centered on appropriate therapies for peripheral neuropathy that could be initially administered in the office and then ultimately in part by the patient at home.

Because of the common links that have been discovered in all the peripheral neuropathies, especially hypoxia or nerve damage, Dr. Phillips and I theorized that anything that can be done to reverse this situation at the cellular level is bound to give the patient improvement. Clinically, this certainly appears to be happening.

We expect the research to tell us much more about why, and also expect to be able to identify precisely what are the most powerful components of this treatment program.

Specifically, when a patient presents for our program and has been proven to be a candidate for treatment after thorough evaluation, manual therapies are applied. The manual therapies may include spinal manipulation, massage, and stretching and exercise therapy. Keep in mind that these therapies are only applied, when indicated, by licensed healthcare professionals and specifically directed towards biomechanical faults. These are identified during the patient's initial physical examination.

Part of the initial assessment of our patients with peripheral neuropathy includes nutrition evaluations. Upon performing the patient's nutritional evaluation, specific dietary supplements may be recommended. We have found in most patients that the application of ReStore, the supplement invented by Dr. Phillips, seems to greatly enhance the treatment program.

Furthermore, other dietary supplements as mentioned earlier, may prove to be very effective as well.

The third part of this 3-part solution for rapid change is the application of the ReBuilder dual-frequency nerve stimulator invented by Dr. David Phillips. The ReBuilder is an amazing device. The ReBuilder supplies simultaneous alternating and direct current. It's important to note that approximately 80,000 of these units have been in use around the world without a single lawsuit or serious adverse incident reported. The treatment units are simple and easy to use.

Why is the ReBuilder unit so effective? The application of neuro-stimulation at the identical frequency that is propagated along the nerve in the human body has been duplicated by Dr. Phillips. The duplication and amplification of this nerve signal seems to enhance and improve—in fact, restore—normal nerve-cell communication.

How is the ReBuilder stimulation administered? The ReBuilder stimulation employed in our offices in the first five weeks is through the application of what Dr. Phillips has called the "wet dual-compartment method." Quite simply, a warm dual-compartment footbath is drawn, which consists of water and the application of some electrolyte solution that helps the conductivity of the electric signal into the tissue. Personally, I like the application of the wet method initially because it gives the nerve path a very wide signal area to travel through. It also has the added benefit of producing vasodilation, or opening up the blood vessels.

In my patients, especially my chemotherapy patients who have had chronic skin and temperature changes, I have found that in just a few treatments we have had amazing restoration of skin temperature and I believe that this is in large part due to the application of the wet method.

Further research will certainly help to illuminate us on exactly why this may be happening.

The administration of the ReBuilder therapy is completely comfortable. You sit in a chair, monitored by a staff person and have complete control of the device at all times. Initially, you may not feel anything at all as the ReBuilder stimulation is applied. After an initial therapy session consisting of 15 minutes of ReBuilder therapy, a subsequent 15-minute session is administered at approximately the same frequency on the next visit. We have had the greatest success by subsequently and very gradually increasing the frequency of ReBuilder therapy until we start to notice a very significant improvement in skin temperature. The patient begins to report some considerable improvement in their symptoms in as little as two weeks after beginning this combined treatment modality.

7

Can't I Treat Myself?

You can treat yourself. However, we have found the vast majority of patients that we treat are far better off having an initial period of supervision. Furthermore, it is our opinion and experience that peripheral neuropathy patients need to be very thoroughly evaluated and monitored by a central treating licensed healthcare professional. This allows the patient to have one person to coordinate their care and ensure that any necessary diagnostic tests that should have been done have been done, and that the patient's other healthcare conditions are fully addressed.

We firmly believe that one of the greatest reasons for our success has been that we insist our patients undergo a five-week clinical trial in the office prior to being discharged with the homecare unit. This trial includes often a nutritional evaluation and extensive clinical baseline and follow-up exams.

We administer con-current manual therapies, prescriptive exercises, nutritional support, communication lines with your other doctors, and really spend the entire 5 weeks educating and training you in all the important factors and co-factors to best insure your recovery of function, and reduction in severity of your symptoms, some of my patients have reported up to 90% improvements, and ***never*** has a compliant patient ever reported less than 20% improvement during the initial period.

It's important to note, most patients have also reported a progressive worsening of their symptoms on the 4-5 years prior to coming under the care with this protocol.

There are circumstances in which patients are unable to attend a clinical trial or are homebound. For those patients, we still recommend professional guidance and evaluations and are going to great lengths through our website http://neuropathydr.com to provide this guidance for these patients. We can even provide telemedicine evaluations when accessible by both parties.

8

What About Insurance in Paying for Care?

The doctors who employ our treatment modalities are very experienced in working with peripheral neuropathy patients. Furthermore, they have gone to great lengths to learn our methods of treatment and will go to great lengths to make your care not only effective but affordable as well.

In many cases, there will be an out-of-pocket cost. But don't forget to use your FSA, HCSA, or simply remember to deduct medical expenditures where applicable. ***This out of pocket expense for a five week clinical trial is often far less than you may already be spending on marginally effective prescription medication.***

There is also the possibility that your insurance company may provide reimbursement for some or all of your care and your doctors good records from your 5 week clinical trial may very well assist you in recovering from your insurance.

9

Finding a Professional to Manage Your Care

Finding a professional trained in our system to manage your care is now easier than ever. We are training doctors and therapists around the world to use this unique system, consisting of the three key components. In my opinion, only those professionals (MD, DC, DO, DPM, PT) with appropriate training are best suited to evaluate and administer this care, because of the vast degree of skills needed in diagnosis, manual therapies, clinical experience as well as nutrition therapies, which many allopathic physicians typically are not trained in.

You can go to http://neuropathydr.com and look for doctors who are well versed or in training with our treatment methodology and our treatment systems. We have very cost effective training and support available for physicians and physical therapists which is expanding exponentially.

10

Conclusion

In conclusion, this book is meant *only* to be an introduction about very successful treatment of a condition that affects many millions of people worldwide. Please understand that should your doctor like detailed clinical information, he or she may contact us at http://neuropathydr.com.

I am very pleased to announce that as more doctors are trained in this system we will be gathering extensive information and expect to publish clinical trials in the not-too-distant future. We also continue to report on a regular basis the case histories, initial presentations, objective findings and the dramatic improvements through the application of our system.

I wish you the very best along your journey. We are here to help you. This book purchase is only a starting point for you, or your loved one.

For further information on getting started in your own neuropathy treatment program, please contact us via the web-form at http://neuropathydr.com.

Epilogue

Fixing HealthCare with Common Sense

What it will finally take is anyone's guess. Our politicians in office are great at talking a good game, but what ultimately it will take is a combination of "Common Sense" (written in 1776 from Founding Father Thomas Paine*) and a return of major corporate ethics, with effective, consumer driven oversight and simplified regulation.

A private, free enterprise system, is the only one most Americans will tolerate. Let's finally put the consumer in charge, just like most auto insurance (except of course in Massachusetts).

The lawmakers should simultaneously expand HSAs (healthcare savings accounts) and FSA (flexible spending accounts) and similar programs and benefits to further breed responsible healthcare consumption.

It is likely the best solution, easiest to implement without burdening us with bigger government.

I say let companies like Geico, Progressive and others that market auto insurance direct to consumers into the ring. Let consumer choice drive them to cut costs by uncoupling dollars from non-benefits payment. Give them simple rules to follow, nationwide, exempt from state lines. This could be huge, and would not take any dismantling of our major delivery systems.

Last I checked, Medicare runs on about 4% administrative overhead, but currently private health insurers are closer to 25%. Much of this goes to the questionably ethical profiteering of extreme proportions, exorbitant salaries for executives and contributes to ridiculously poor provider reimbursements.

And, *how about* adding return of premium benefits to reward the healthiest while not penalizing the seriously ill. This is a tremendously powerful idea that would reap huge benefits for the consumer. It's already done with disability and some other types of insurance and mutual insurance companies regularly pay dividends to payees.

So, Lets make sure that some of insurance premium dollars can be returned if consumers work to stay healthy.

Let's also finally de-link health insurance from employers and employment benefits once and for all. This has been an absolute catastrophe. Even the Boston Globe recently acknowledged this. The extreme burden on US businesses of all sizes from health care premiums is well known. The trickle down benefits to business, like the automakers, municipalities and others could also be a huge economic stimulus.

Uncoupling health insurance benefits from employment would make consumers ultimately more fiscally savvy and responsible. This could quite likely increase their wages simultaneously as employees would now purchase all benefits outside of their work. Uncle Sam can help with deductibility and tax exemptions, maybe larger in the beginning to help foster the transition.

I also believe that there should be real consumer dollars available for CAM (Complimentary and Alternative Medicine) that can be used in the treatment of our most common and non-life threatening disorders especially **if** the consumer does not utilize more expensive traditional pathways for the same condition. Back pain and headaches are two very real examples that both happen to be still the most common reasons for doctor's visits, and are at least in part linked to stress and unhealthy lifestyles.

This mechanism alone would foster consumer education to choose their own healthcare pathways with taking an additional financial hit in addition to premiums.

Any effective system must simultaneously provide equitable reimbursement and other incentives to all licensed doctors of all disciplines as well as ancillary providers for our society to keep great healthcare providers in the system.

This must include simplified reimbursement schedules, equal across the professions for identical procedures. I strongly favor a diagnosis-based system with utilization review only for those cases outlying the norms. This could be a technological piece of cake with a national electronic healthcare database for all Americans.

Of course, there are other issues that need to be simultaneously addressed. These include malpractice provisions (some experts suggest in a separate healthcare "court" in addition to capped awards). Better awareness of poor outcomes vs. malpractice by society at large would really help as well.

Drug costs, competition and widespread availability of tested alternatives to prescription drugs all need to be handled. Again, a consumer driven Wal-Mart type of distribution may be what already does it.

So, how can we help? Let's make sure we educate ourselves first and foremost as to what's wrong with our current system and push our lawmakers toward better consumer choices. Take a real hard look at their differences on these topics when you vote and support any politician, as some are huge. Let your friends and family know who these consumer friendly elected officials are in your area are too.

Utilize cost effective preventive screenings and advocate the same for all our families. Lets make sure we teach our kids all the rewards of better health choices like non-smoking, stress management, diabetes prevention, relationship choices including illicit drugs and sexual behavior, and permanent weight control.

How it will all turn out is anybodies guess. I continue to be as vocal about these issues with my patients and community, and urge you to do the same.

Not Unlike Thomas Paine did over 200 years ago.

*(*Society in every state is a blessing, but Government, even in its best state, is but a necessary evil; in its worst state an intolerable one: for when we suffer, or are exposed to the same miseries BY A GOVERNMENT, which we might expect in a country WITHOUT GOVERNMENT, our calamity is heightened by reflecting that we furnish the means by which we suffer.)*

John P Hayes Jr. DC, MS, DABCO

Author of "Living and Practicing by Design" September 2008, and "Beating Neuropathy" January 2010.

LaVergne, TN USA
14 July 2010
189406LV00001B/1/P